HOUSING
OPTIONS FOR
OLDER PEOPLE

DAVID BOOKBINDER

Acknowledgements

I would like to thank a number of people whose comments on specific sections of the booklet were extremely helpful: Chris Cloke, Lee McManus and Rose Moreno of Age Concern England; Melinda McGarry of Age Concern Scotland; Martyn Letall of Shelter; Mike McQueen of Nationwide Building Society; Jane Minter of the National Federation of Housing Associations; Geoff Randall and Karen Smith of SHAC and John Stanford of RADAR.

My thanks also to Iris Searle for typing the manuscript and especially to Nancy Tuft for her unfussy but highly competent editing.

© Age Concern England, May 1987
Bernard Sunley House
60 Pitcairn Road
Mitcham, Surrey CR4 3LL.

ISBN 0-86242-055-5

Editor Nancy Tuft
Design Eugenie Dodd
Production Joyce O'Shaughnessy
Typeset by Parchment (Oxford) Ltd.
Printed by Eyre & Spottiswoode, The Grosvenor Press, Portsmouth

Contents

Author's introduction

In writing this booklet I am not suggesting that people should change their housing circumstances just because they happen to have reached retirement age. Many older people are perfectly happy to carry on just as they are, fortunate enough to be living in a good home in the area of their choice. But many people for very good reasons are not at all satisfied with their housing situation and are seeking to improve it so that they can spend their later years as comfortably as possible.

The book seeks to look at all the options open to older people, but at the same time attempts to give a realistic indication of how easy or otherwise each option may be to pursue successfully. Older people do not have an unlimited range of options to choose from. Sadly, a combination of circumstances means that many people have a very limited choice, but this book can at least ensure that they have looked at all the possible courses of action.

During the last seven or eight years Government spending on housing has been cut by over 60% in real terms, far more than any other area of public expenditure. Despite the fact that many housing providers such as councils and housing associations try to give priority to provision for elderly people, the effects of the cuts cannot be avoided. There is relatively little rented housing being built, fewer repairs being carried out to council houses, and less money available to home owners wanting to repair their homes. All this is at a time when the number of people over 75 is increasing rapidly.

The booklet looks at housing options for older people who have already reached retirement age or who will be doing so in the next year or two, and who are by and large fairly independent. It does not look in detail at domiciliary care services or at residential and nursing homes, although throughout the book there are references for people wanting more detailed information on these particular options.

The booklet is aimed at older people throughout the UK: variations in Scotland are mentioned in the text where appropriate, and readers in Northern Ireland may already know that the Northern Ireland Housing Executive (rather than local councils) is responsible for most state housing matters.

At various points in the text there are references to housing costs for which assistance is available in certain circumstances. This information relates to welfare benefits available before April 1988. At that time the social security system will be radically changed and you should check then that you have up to date details of the new regulations.

Nowhere in the booklet do I indicate what are the *best* housing options, as that is impossible. I have given details of options that may be available so that you can make an informed choice, depending on your particular circumstances.

David Bookbinder
April 1987

1·STAY AT HOME OR MOVE?

In the next few pages we look at some of the questions worth asking yourself if you are unsure whether to stay at home or move. Many of you will feel there is no decision to make because you have already made up your mind.

Some of you will want to stay where you are, in which case you will need to find out whether any problems at home can be resolved, for example the need for repair work.

Others will already be keen to move, either within the same locality but into more suitable housing, or to another area altogether, possibly to be nearer relatives and perhaps into more suitable housing at the same time.

Some of the points in this section will probably seem pretty obvious, but Age Concern's experience is that far too many older people make big decisions about their future without thinking things through sufficiently carefully.

Thinking early   For those who are unsure what to do the importance of thinking ahead cannot be over-emphasised. Moving home never happens quickly and needs careful planning, and if you own your home and want to stay there, you may have the chance to get some improvement or repair work carried out before you stop working and your income decreases.

Whether you are thinking of moving or staying put, a delay in taking any action at all is likely to lessen the options open to you. Some early steps may be well worth taking, such as applying to get on council or housing association waiting lists, or enquiring about home improvement grants. Neither commits you to any definite decision at this stage but will at least help keep your options open for later.

Thinking early should not mean thinking hurriedly. Often older people who have recently been bereaved, particularly widows who have just lost their husbands, want to move home as soon as possible. At such a difficult time, this is understandable and in some cases may well eventually turn out to be the best option. But there is a real danger of making a panic decision without first allowing time to adjust to a new way of life.

Conversely some people tend to stay on indefinitely in an unsuitable house solely for memory's sake. What was once an ideal family house may well be expensive to heat and difficult to maintain on a single pension and may be inappropriate accommodation for an older person living alone today.

1·1 Thinking of staying at home?

The main questions for people thinking of staying at home include:

- Do you like your home, is it convenient for your needs and in reasonable repair?
- Can you afford the running costs?
- Do you like the area?
- Are you near relatives and friends?
- If you need help with tasks such as gardening, decorating or shopping, is such assistance available?

Council, housing association and private tenants Sadly they have less control over their housing situation than do most home owners but one or two further questions may still be worth asking:

- What are the chances of any necessary repairs or modernisation being carried out? Unfortunately they may be rather slim: even though many councils and housing associations are concentrating their resources on maintenance rather than on new building, the amount being spent on repairs is still a long way below what is required. In privately rented housing getting the landlord to carry out repairs or improvements is frequently very difficult.

- What is happening to the area you live in? Is it improving or deteriorating?

Home owners Owner-occupiers can consider a number of factors:

- Do any minor or major repairs need doing, or might they be needed in the foreseeable future? A lack of knowledge of house maintenance often makes people reluctant or unable to recognise the need for repair work. Anxiety about financing repairs and the problem of finding a decent and reliable builder may also deter people from taking any action.

- Could the home be converted or adapted to make life more comfortable? Putting in a downstairs bathroom or a hand-rail on the stairs are just two examples.

- What would it cost to repair, improve or adapt your home and is there any help available, in terms of both specialist advice and finance?

- If you have a garden, is it too much to cope with? Can you get any help with it?

Later sections in the booklet will offer guidance on these points.

1·2 Thinking of moving?

The pros and cons of moving are different for everyone, depending on their present housing circumstances. You will see that the list of possible disadvantages is quite long, but rather than aiming to deter you from moving, its purpose is to urge you to consider all the factors carefully.

Possible advantages of moving

- It could be to better and more suitable housing, probably smaller than your current home and easier to look after. Hopefully it will be less costly to heat as well.
- It could be to a nicer or more familiar area.
- It could be much nearer to family or friends.
- It could be nearer to a local community, shops, transport and other services if these are what you are missing now.

Possible disadvantages of moving

- Even if you are moving near to relatives, how many other people do you know in the new area? You may miss friends you used to have.
- If you are a couple do you *both* have relatives or friends in the new area? No-one wants to think about it, but what if one of you dies and the surviving partner knows hardly anyone in the area? It will not be easy to return to where you used to live, and could be almost impossible if you want to get back into rented accommodation there.
- Although you may be moving nearer to relatives, is there a chance that they themselves might move from that area in the future? People do not stay in the same job in the same place all their working lives.
- You may have to get used to an unfamiliar area and only then realise that you miss your former neighbourhood. Good shops may be further away than you want, and you should bear in mind that many small, local shops are closing down nowadays.
- You could find that public transport services are already poor or will deteriorate in the near future. Deregulation of services now means that a number of unprofitable routes may disappear. The services may not be the same all year round, and you may find them more expensive than you are used to. You cannot take it for granted that there will be any concessionary fares. These issues may seem unimportant if you have a car but will you always be a driver?
- How near will you be to a post office, library, pub and other facilities? Will there be a doctor, dentist, optician, chiropodist

etc. within convenient distance? How far away is the nearest hospital?

- If now or in the future you need social services assistance such as home help or meals on wheels, you may not be able to obtain these automatically in your new area. You may also find that there are no lunch clubs or day centres nearby.
- If you are moving to a smaller home you are unlikely to be able to keep all your furniture and possessions.
- Removal fees will need to be paid and if you are buying and selling, the estate agent's and solicitor's fees as well.

2·MOVING HOME

2·1 What type of housing do you want?

Even though you may not be altogether happy with your present accommodation, you may not yet have thought carefully about what sort of housing you really want. It may be that you are quite happy with the type of housing you currently occupy and that you just want to move to another area. But many older people do find their present accommodation far from suitable.

You may like to use any opportunities which arise to look around at different types of accommodation. For example, you can visit friends or acquaintances already living in sheltered accommodation, or take advantage of private developers' show houses which are open to view. You may have no intention of buying, but at least you will get some idea of what is currently available and you can make useful comparisons.

In looking at special housing for older people the impression is often given that sheltered housing is what everyone looking for alternative accommodation wants. On the contrary: older people often want something smaller (but not too small), easier to look after and cheaper to heat. The presence of a warden is not a key factor for many people. For some it is not even necessary to have ground-floor accommodation, although for a large number this is what they want most of all.

Special housing without a warden

Many councils and housing associations have rented housing which is either purpose-built or converted especially for older people, although there is no warden. Its design and location should mean the accommodation is particularly suitable for older people, but because there are numerous interpretations of what is appropriate, this type of housing varies enormously, and you should find out exactly what special features a particular property has. Also many private companies now sell specially designed housing without warden support.

Sheltered housing

In recent years the demand for sheltered housing has been very heavy and there is no sign of this changing. Coming at the same time as Government cuts in the public sector house building programme, this heavy demand now means that moving to rented sheltered housing can be very difficult, and in same areas almost impossible. The scarcity of vacancies for sheltered housing makes it especially important that you know exactly what this type of accommodation consists of, as you obviously don't want to waste time considering housing that would not be suitable.

In many areas – particularly in the South – it is now possible to buy sheltered housing if you are fortunate enough to be able to consider this option (see page 37).

Most conventional sheltered housing (sometimes called warden-assisted or warden-controlled housing) is a development of self-contained one or two-bedroom flats, normally between 25 and 40, with a resident warden and an alarm system in each flat for use in an emergency. Sometimes wardens are known as resident managers or by a similar job title. Some sheltered schemes are made up of bungalows. Meals are not normally provided for residents, who have their own kitchen facilities. The external maintenance, insurance, gardening and window-cleaning etc. are not the responsibility of residents.

Sheltered housing is generally intended for fairly active,

independent people, even though some councils allocate it on the basis of medical circumstances. So if you are happy to go on doing your own shopping and cooking but feel you need the security of warden cover, it may be that sheltered housing would be appropriate.

What does the warden do? Most wardens act as 'good neighbours', keeping a discreet eye on residents and calling for appropriate help in an emergency. The warden may call on residents each day just to check that all is well, but it is important to note that she/he is not there to help with shopping, cooking, cleaning or personal tasks such as dressing, bathing or nursing.

There is no reason why people in sheltered housing cannot apply for domiciliary assistance from social services such as home help or meals on wheels if available, and, if you wish, the warden may be able to arrange this. But if you need any significant degree of personal care sheltered housing is unlikely to be the right option.

Other features of sheltered housing These normally include a guest room, common room and laundry facilities. The size of individual flats or bungalows varies, with some schemes (particularly older ones) having bedsitters. Even some of the newer one-bedroom flats are very small. The amount of available storage space also varies.

In many but not all sheltered housing schemes there is a lounge for use by the residents and there is often a residents' social committee to organise activities and outings. The extent to which residents socialise with each other varies from scheme to scheme and of course everyone can choose for themselves how much they mix with others. Going into sheltered housing certainly doesn't guarantee that you'll never feel lonely, but there should normally be plenty of opportunities to talk with other people, strike up friendships and feel that you are part of a community.

Pets Some schemes do not permit pets at all, whilst others will allow you to bring in your existing pet but not to replace it when it dies. There may in some cases be no restriction if your home has direct access to a garden area, but in many sheltered flats there is no such access.

Gardens Although many people may be glad to get away from a garden, some schemes have garden areas which residents may be able to help look after. Schemes made up of bungalows are more likely to have small individual gardens.

Abbeyfield houses

Local Abbeyfield societies nationwide manage over 900 large houses, in each of which between seven and nine elderly people have their own bed-sitting room with their own furniture. Residents come together for the main meals of the day, which are prepared by the resident housekeeper. The provision of meals means that the weekly charge is much higher than sheltered housing, but people on a very low income should be able to obtain some assistance through supplementary or housing benefit.

Abbeyfield's supportive houses, as they are called, tend to be popular because the support includes not just the provision of meals but also a family-type atmosphere. At the same time it is possible for the residents to retain some privacy. The supportive houses are normally intended for fairly active, independent older people.

Some local Abbeyfield societies now run special extra-care schemes providing a much higher level of care than is available in their usual supportive houses.

Abbeyfield residents are considered to be licensees and do not therefore have the security of tenure enjoyed by most housing association tenants. It would be wise to obtain independent advice about your rights before going into an Abbeyfield house.

*Details of your nearest Abbeyfield house can be obtained from the head office of the **Abbeyfield Society**, 186-192 Darkes Lane, Potters Bar, Hertfordshire EN6 1AB. Tel: 0707 44845.*

Almshouses

Almshouses date back many centuries, having been provided by landowners and other benefactors for elderly people in need. Most have been fully modernised and there are also newly-built flats and bungalows, some of which are warden-assisted. Almshouses are provided rent and rates free, but there may be a weekly maintenance contribution (at a level authorised by the Charity Commissioners) towards the upkeep. This contribution is treated as rent for which supplementary benefit or housing benefit can usually be paid to those who qualify.

In legal terms almshouse residents are beneficiaries of the Trust governing that particular almshouse charity. As such they do not have security of tenure, but the terms of occupation are established by a letter of appointment and residents considered to be licensees. As the rights of licensees can sometimes be unclear, you should seek advice from a solicitor, Citizens Advice Bureau or housing advice centre before becoming an almshouse resident.

Each group of almshouses is managed by its own trustees, and standards of provision and management vary considerably. Many almshouses are restricted to particular applicants, in accordance with the original benefactor's wishes.

Information on almshouses can be obtained from the **National Association of Almshouses**, *Billingbear Lodge, Wokingham, Berkshire RG11 5RU. Tel: 0344 52922.*

Housing with care services provided

Some councils and housing associations (but only one or two private companies) have a form of sheltered housing with additional services such as meals and higher staffing levels. The aim of these schemes, as with normal sheltered housing, is to enable residents to retain independence as far as possible, whilst receiving help with domestic duties or in some cases with personal tasks. Nursing is not provided in these schemes.

This housing is sometimes called 'very sheltered housing' or 'extra-care sheltered housing' and is intended for people who find that although they need more support than sheltered housing usually offers, they do not need to go into a residential home. Unfortunately there is not much extra-care sheltered housing available and if you cannot get into this type of accommodation you should always check on what additional help might be available to assist you at home, both in terms of domiciliary services and help with improving or adapting your home.

Residential and nursing homes

If you need a high degree of personal care which cannot be provided in your own home, it is likely that you will need to consider going into residential care, although you would of course need to discuss this with your doctor, social worker and family. Local councils have a limited number of residential homes and there are many which are run privately or by voluntary organisations. Standards of care and accommodation vary greatly, although all private and voluntary homes caring for more than three people must be registered with the local authority. The social services department will have a list of homes in the area. You should never consider a home that is not registered, nor one that you have not first visited. A trial stay enables you to get the feel of a home and to find out if it really provides a satisfactory standard of care.

If you require the availability of 24-hour nursing care, a nursing home is likely to be necessary. Almost all are privately run and must be registered with the District Health Authority, which will have a list of homes in the area.

Some special accommodation agencies are listed in Age Concern England's fact sheet No. 29 *Finding Residential and Nursing Home Accommodation* available free on receipt of a $9\frac{1}{2}$" x $6\frac{1}{2}$" SAE from the Information and Policy Department. This fact sheet also gives advice on how to decide which home is best for your needs.

Information on the system of charges for residential and nursing care, and on how DHSS assistance is calculated, is contained in two other fact sheets from Age Concern England:

No. 10 *Local Authorities and Residential Care* and No. 11
Supplementary Benefit for Residential and Nursing Homes.
These are available free on receipt of a 9½" x 6½" SAE from the
Information and Policy Department. It should be noted that
the entire social security system changes in April 1988, when
updated fact sheets will be produced.

Further advice on seeking residential and nursing homes can be
obtained from **Counsel and Care for the Elderly**, *131 Middlesex*
Street, London E1 7JF. Tel: 01 621 1624.

Retirement centres

Age Concern receives many enquiries from people who have
read or heard about retirement centres, consisting of a special
housing scheme accompanied by an on-site restaurant, post
office, shops and a medical centre. Such projects are not
common in this country and are not therefore a realistic
housing option. The high cost of providing such facilities and
the desire among housing providers to avoid isolating elderly
people in one place are just two reasons for this. Where such
retirement villages have been built in other countries, such as
in the United States, they are often very expensive to live in.

Housing for elderly people with disabilities

Most local councils and some housing associations have a
limited amount of 'mobility' and 'wheelchair' housing.

Mobility housing is often little different from ordinary housing
except that it has no steps or stairs and should be in a
convenient location near to shops etc. It may be suitable for
people who are not confined to a wheelchair inside the house,
even if they use one outdoors.

Wheelchair housing on the other hand is purpose-built and
has a number of special features such as wide doorways, level
or ramped access instead of steps, as well as specially
designed bathrooms and toilets, and kitchens with electric
sockets and working surfaces at a suitable height.

Much of the sheltered housing provided by local authorities
and housing associations is designed as mobility housing but

some schemes include dwellings designed for people who use wheelchairs. As well as contacting the council you should also write to the appropriate regional office of the **Housing Corporation** to see if there are any housing associations in your area with housing for people with disabilities.

Very little of the sheltered housing being built for sale to elderly people is designed to wheelchair standards, but it may be worth contacting developers who are planning or building in the area to ask if alterations could be made to the basic design of a flat or bungalow for a committed purchaser. Alternatively you may be able to buy a suitable flat or house and adapt it, in which case you should check whether there is any help available through improvement grants, the social services department or building society loans (see page 50).

A booklet entitled Buying or Adapting a House or Flat – A Consumer Guide for Disabled People is available price £1 (incl. p + p) from Centre on Environment for the Handicapped, 35 Great Smith Street, London SW1P 3BJ. Tel: 01 222 7980.

Housing for elderly people from ethnic minorities

Research has suggested that many elderly people from numerous different ethnic minorities would prefer to spend their later years largely with people from their own culture. Sadly, not only are there very few council or housing association schemes for elderly people from ethnic minorities, but most existing housing provision for elderly people is unsuitable, partly because of its design and location and mainly because it ignores the special social, cultural, dietary and religious needs of people from ethnic minorities.

Your local housing advice centre or Community Relations Council should have details of any special housing schemes which might meet your particular needs.

Mobile homes

Some older people, including home owners who cannot afford to buy new property after selling up, consider the possibility of buying a mobile home (also known as a park home). If you are contemplating this option you should be sure that you will feel comfortable in what may well be a very confined amount of space, and you should not make your decision on the basis of a week's holiday in a mobile home.

Furthermore, although the 1983 Mobile Homes Act brought certain improvements for mobile home residents, there are still a number of pitfalls to watch out for:

- The purchase price can be very high. Larger building societies now have the power to lend up to £10,000 for mobile homes but most do not do this. The only other source for a loan is a finance company who will charge a very high interest rate.

- You will also have to pay rates and a weekly rent for your pitch. Rates can be very high, particularly in holiday areas; pitch rents also can be substantial, and subject to annual increases.

- Some mobile homes can be expensive to heat, as insulation is often poor. Insulation standards for new mobile homes are now much improved.

- Although you are a home owner you are, in effect, renting your pitch and the use of the common parts of the park from the site owner. Your rights and those of the site owner are governed by the content of the written agreement that you must have. It is crucial that this agreement is checked by a solicitor before you agree to buy.

- You should also try to check (perhaps by asking other residents on the park) that the site owner is reasonable, as he or she could cause problems for the new mobile home owner.

- If you want to sell up you must pay a commission (10% at April 1987) to the site owner and this is quite a high sum. Site owners also have the right to refuse to give consent for you to sell to a particular purchaser, although they must give good reasons.

A booklet called *Mobile Homes – A Guide for Residents and Site Owners* (Housing Booklet No. 16) is available free from Citizens Advice Bureaux and advice centres.

*In order to check on what factors you should consider when contemplating the purchase of a mobile home you can send a 9½" x 6½" SAE for a very useful guide, obtainable from the **Mobile Homes Unit, Shelter**, 88 Old Street, London EC1V 9AX.*

Moving abroad

The possible pitfalls of moving home already mentioned on page 12 become even more important to consider if you are thinking of moving abroad, either permanently or just for part of the year, for example winter. As well as checking with the DHSS on how your pension entitlement will be affected, and with the Inland Revenue on your tax situation, you should check in particular on what health care, if any, is available and how much it would cost: few other countries have the equivalent of the National Health Service. If you are considering a move abroad you should contact the appropriate embassy and find out as much information as possible.

Returning from abroad

A substantial number of people who moved abroad at some earlier point in the past either before or after retirement are now returning to spend the rest of their later life in the U.K. These older people, however, now face major problems regarding accommodation unless they have considerable capital assets. The chronic shortage of rented housing means that it may not be possible for any council or housing association to rehouse them. For anyone returning from abroad, however long they may previously have lived in the U.K., the chances are that they would have to seek accommodation in the private sector, either for rent or purchase, depending on their financial situation.

Moving in with relatives

It is not easy to advise on the pros and cons of going to live with relatives, as so much depends on the particular people and circumstances involved. There are many factors to take into account and if you are seriously considering this option you may wish to obtain Age Concern England's booklet *Sharing Your Home* available after October 1987 from the Marketing Department. Please check the price before ordering.

For many families everything works out fine, but in some cases it can create tensions, with both the elderly person and the family usually wanting to retain their privacy and independence. The situation could be especially difficult if there are children, most of whom understandably want to spend some of their spare time being noisy! You would also have to look very carefully at whether the design and layout of your relatives' home are suitable for you now, and in particular at whether they would still be suitable if you were to become less mobile in the future.

It is most important to consider the financial implications of moving in with relatives. If you have previously been living in your own home and receiving financial assistance with rent and rates, it is unlikely you will receive this help once you are living with relatives, regardless of the fact that your income will presumably be the same. If you receive supplementary pension your weekly scale rate will be far less than if you were living in your own home, although you would receive an allowance for housing expenses (£3.90 at April 1987).

Many elderly people living with relatives wish to pay something towards accommodation and food bills but you should never move in with relatives on the assumption you will be able to pay them and then claim supplementary or housing benefit. Even if you have your own self-contained flatlet within the family's house, it is not likely that help will be given with rent or rates.

Other points to consider include arrangements for meals. Some elderly people sharing with relatives have their own cooking facilities for snacks and mid-day meals, and join the family for main meals in the evenings and at weekends. Alternatively, if as often happens, all your meals are prepared for you, you may have to get used to eating at times which suit the whole family. If your relatives are working full-time, this could mean eating later in the evening than you would otherwise do.

How easy would it be for you to have visitors? You might be more reluctant to ask your own friends to call, particularly if a lack of space leaves you with less privacy than you would like.

'Granny annexes'

Granny flats or annexes, as they are often called, may be an option some elderly people and their families wish to consider, although at the present time it is not one that many people pursue. Living with relatives – and yet living separately – is an ideal situation for some but an uneasy compromise for others. Many understandably dislike the idea of living in an extension tacked on to the side of the house or in a portakabin or prefab at the bottom of the garden.

Such accommodation would have to be built and funded privately: there is no special financial assistance available and planning permission would also be required. Again, such an arrangement may not normally be considered as living in a separate household and you would therefore be unlikely to get help with rent and rates.

If you are uncertain of what your benefits situation would be if you go to live with relatives, you should seek advice from a welfare rights advice centre or Citizens Advice Bureau.

2·2 Achieving a move – to rented housing in the same area

By and large, looking for privately rented housing should be a last resort, and you should always obtain advice from a Citizens Advice Bureau or housing advice centre before signing any tenancy, as you could risk accepting an agreement which leaves you with few rights. If you do move to privately rented housing and your rent is higher than before, you should check with the local council's housing benefit section to see whether you are entitled to any help with the rent and rates.

Otherwise the main sources of rented accommodation are the council and local housing associations.

Applying for council housing

Whether you are seeking conventional accommodation or special housing, the local council's housing department will be the first port of call. Unfortunately, as so little new council housing has been built and many existing homes sold to sitting tenants in recent years, waiting lists are normally very long. Councils all have their own policies for allocating housing but in any area you are likely to be competing not only with other elderly people in desperate need of rehousing but also with young people, families and homeless people. The waiting list for sheltered housing is often particularly long.

Many councils in England and Wales feel unable to consider home owners for rehousing into rented accommodation, as priority is given to people with no capital assets. This can be harsh for those home owners whose properties would not bring sufficient to enable another purchase to be made. There may be other options for older people in this predicament (see page 32) but it is an unfortunate trap in which to be caught.

Applying for a transfer If you are already a council tenant and wish to move within the same area you should contact the housing department to request a transfer either to more suitable accommodation and/or to a different part of the locality. As well as the difficulties caused by long waiting lists, many council areas are now very large, and even if you are made an offer it may be for housing in an area with which you are not familiar.

Many councils allow tenants to exchange with each other, but this is of course dependent on your home and the area being desirable enough to attract interest.

Housing associations

In most areas there are a number of housing associations providing rented accommodation for people with special needs, including older people. These associations are funded mainly by grants from the **Housing Corporation**, a body set up by the Government and local authorities. Not all the accommodation allocated to older people is sheltered, but most is likely at least to be ground-floor and should be conveniently located. As housing associations are relatively recent, compared with local councils, much of their housing for older people is purpose-built.

Housing associations do not provide anywhere near the same amount of housing as councils, and because they have not been able to build as much as they would have liked in recent years, due again to Government spending cuts, their waiting lists can also be very long. One point to note is that many associations take 50% (and in some cases 100%) of their applicants direct from the local council, for which you would normally have to be high on the council waiting list. Also, some associations may not be able to consider applications from home owners, or may not consider them a priority.

Your local council or housing advice centre should have details of housing associations in the area, as should your regional **Housing Corporation** office. Also Age Concern England has a list of housing associations for each county in England as well as each London Borough. Send a large SAE to the Information and Policy Department, stating which area you are interested in.

2·3 Achieving a move – to rented housing in a different area

Moving to rented accommodation in a different area is something many older people wish to do, particularly those who want to be nearer relatives. Unfortunately the acute shortage of rented accommodation has led many councils and housing associations to adopt strict policies on the allocation of housing to people from other areas. It can be especially difficult if you need sheltered housing.

Council housing

The first step is to approach the housing department of the council in the area you wish to move to. You may well find that the council has residence restrictions, for example requiring that applicants must have been living in the area for a specified period (say two years) immediately prior to applying. This is mainly because councils with only a limited number of lettings each year feel they must give priority to people living locally. It means that even if in the past you spent many years or perhaps most of your life in that area, you are still required to return and live there for the specified period before you can be considered for rehousing. In practice this is unlikely to be possible for most people.

Additionally, home owners may find that the council cannot consider them at all, so if you want to move to rented housing in a new area *and* you are a home owner you could lose out on both counts.

Often when you apply to another council they will consider you only if the council in your current area is prepared to nominate you. You may find that in order for your council to do this you must be a council tenant or high on the waiting list. This can be frustrating for people who are not on their own council's waiting list because they have never wanted rehousing in their current area.

Some councils have other reciprocal arrangements to rehouse a certain number of applicants into the other council's area, though the number of people achieving a move in this way is very limited.

Almost all councils participate in the **National Mobility Scheme** introduced by the Government to help people with a pressing social need to move to another area. You should ask your local council about this, but sadly, each council makes available only a tiny proportion of its annual vacancies for letting under this scheme. You do not necessarily have to be a council tenant to apply, but you can only seek a move under the scheme if the council where you currently live accepts your application.

On the other hand *any* council tenant can attempt to move via the **Tenants Exchange Scheme** on his or her own initiative. This scheme enables one tenant to swap homes with another tenant living in a different area, including Wales and Scotland. The scheme is also open to tenants wanting to move to or from – but not within – Northern Ireland. Obviously the scheme is worth considering only if your current home and the area are reasonably desirable, for which reason it is not a realistic option for many tenants in poor housing.

*A leaflet entitled **Tenants Exchange Scheme** can be obtained from your council housing department or Citizens Advice Bureau, or from **T.E.S.**, P.O. Box 170, London SW1P 3PX.*

You may wish to try advertising in local newspapers in the area you wish to move to, and there is also a private exchange bureau called **Locatex**, which offers to help council and housing association tenants who wish to move to another area, covering England, Wales and Scotland. A one-off fee of £7 (as at April 1987) is payable.

*Their address is **Locatex Bureau**, P.O. Box I, March, Cambridgeshire PE15 8HJ. Tel: 0354 54050.*

Housing associations

Some housing associations also have allocations policies which require that you already reside in the area, although others will consider applicants who have strong ties with the area, such as having close relatives there. As already mentioned, there are numerous competing demands for housing association accommodation and in many cases vacancies arise infrequently. Again you may find some associations unable to consider applications from home owners. For details of how to find out about housing associations go back to page 28.

If you are already a housing association tenant but wish to move to another area, ask your association if they have any suitable housing in your preferred area. Also, if you live within a 100-mile radius of London you should ask your association whether it participates in **HALO** (Housing Associations Liaison Office), a mobility scheme for housing association tenants, through which they might be able to nominate you to another housing association.

2·4 If you become homeless

If for any reason you face the possibility of losing your home, a particular problem for private tenants, you should contact a housing advice centre, Citizens Advice Bureau, law centre, solicitor, or your regional **Shelter Housing Aid Centre**. It would also be advisable to contact the local council's housing department too. Your rights will depend largely on the nature of your tenancy, but almost invariably you will be advised to stay put and not to sign anything. The landlord is likely to have to go through a number of formal procedures if he wants you to leave. Hopefully the council will also be able to give you some indication of your position should the landlord eventually succeed in gaining possession of the property.

The threat of eviction by a private landlord is by no means the only potential cause of homelessness. Often an older person has been living for some time with friends, possibly a family who are now planning to move elsewhere. Someone may in the past have entered into some kind of home sharing agreement based on companionship but which has no proper legal or financial basis. If circumstances change, if they quarrel or one falls ill or dies, then the other can face serious problems, especially if the property has to be sold and he or she has no legal claim. Age Concern hears of many cases where lonely people have sunk their savings in this way.

People of pensionable age who become homeless through no fault of their own will normally be eligible for rehousing by the local council (but not by any other council) under the Housing (Homeless Persons) Act 1977, although you should take nothing for granted. Having to vacate tied accommodation is a common example of 'unintentional homelessness'. The above Act does not apply in Northern Ireland.

Councils cannot normally rehouse you *before* you are actually made homeless, although once this has happened you should be offered temporary accommodation whilst the council is examining your situation. Obviously this can be a very worrying time and you should always seek advice.

2·5 Options for people with limited capital

One of the most unfortunate aspects of the current housing situation is the lack of a broad range of options for older people whose capital is insufficient to enable an outright purchase to be made. Many people live in old housing which would not sell for a particularly good price, and for those wishing to move further South the situation is particularly difficult because of the huge differences in house prices. The few options that are available for people with limited capital are listed here.

Shared ownership

A small number of councils and housing associations run shared ownership schemes where you part-buy and part-rent a property. Some other organisations such as building societies may now be developing shared ownership schemes. As an example, you may buy half with your capital sum and pay rent on the other half. You own your share on the basis of a long lease. If at any stage you are able to increase the purchased share this should be possible. Your local council housing department or housing advice centre should be able to advise whether there are any schemes locally, and the regional office of the **Housing Corporation** should have details of any housing associations running shared ownership schemes. There is a Housing Corporation leaflet called *Shared Ownership* describing how these schemes are run.

Special leasehold schemes

Some housing associations run special **Leasehold Schemes for the Elderly (LSE)** where in most cases you buy at 70% of the normal purchase price and receive back 70% of its value at the time you sell. The schemes are almost always sheltered, and priority may be given to people who either live in the area or have strong ties such as having close relatives there.

Once you have bought your 70% share of the lease, you will

then have to pay a regular service charge each month for the employment of the warden and services such as maintenance, cleaning, gardening etc. You will also have your own rates, water rates and fuel bills to pay, so before committing yourself to one of these schemes you should be sure that your income will be sufficient.

Although these special leasehold schemes are run by housing associations and not by private developers, there are still a number of important factors worth checking up on beforehand and some of these points are highlighted on page 37. The *Buyer's Guide to Sheltered Housing* covers all the points in detail, and is available price £1 (incl. p + p) from Age Concern England's Marketing Department.

The council housing department or housing advice centre should have details of any local schemes, as should your **Housing Corporation** regional office. Age Concern England's fact sheet No. 24 *Housing Schemes for Elderly People Where a Capital Sum is Required* also contains addresses and is available free on receipt of a 9½" x 6½" SAE from the Information and Policy Department.

Loan-stock or investment schemes

A few housing trusts and charitable organisations run loan-stock schemes, sometimes called investment schemes, where an interest-free loan is paid in return for housing, normally sheltered. The size of the loan varies from scheme to scheme. When you leave you receive back the sum you originally paid, without interest. There will, though, be certain deductions (eg for administering the re-sale) and there could be restrictions governing when you actually receive the money after leaving: in some schemes this will not be until the property is re-occupied.

You will also have to pay a monthly service charge and this may be very high. Some organisations (mainly trusts and charities) running these schemes leave much to be desired in terms of their management ability and you should ensure you obtain sound legal advice before committing yourself.

Details of some loan-stock schemes are included in the Age Concern England fact sheet No. 24, mentioned in the preceding section.

Buying sheltered housing at a discount

Some developers building sheltered housing for sale run special schemes whereby the property is offered at a discount. Sometimes the buyer can choose between paying the full price or buying at a discount. The terms of any such scheme should be examined very carefully, as they often involve giving up some or even all of the future appreciation in value.

For example, there may be schemes with the option of paying only 80% of the full price, in which case you should receive 80% of its value at the time you sell. However, another case involving the same discount – for example buying for £40,000 instead of the full price of £50,000 – could mean you receiving back only £40,000 when you eventually sell, even if by then the property is worth, say, £70,000 or more. There is nothing wrong with such schemes providing that the conditions are made clear from the outset.

In the near future there is likely to be an increase in the number of finance companies offering to help older people buy sheltered housing at a discount. These companies do not build housing themselves: once you have selected a property to buy you ask the developer if you can make the purchase through the special terms offered by one of these finance companies. Often where a developer has already linked up with a finance company offering such a discount, it will seem to all intents and purposes that the developer is actually offering the discount directly.

In these schemes the size of the discount is dependent on your age, sex and whether you are single or a couple. The older you are the bigger the discount; men receive more than women and single people more than couples as the discounts are based on average life expectancies. The main feature to note is that once you have bought at a discount the entire value of the property passes to the company on your death. Sometimes the sales literature does not immediately make this clear. For example it might state that in return for obtaining a discount you receive a 'life-share' in the property. Your solicitor should of course ensure that you are fully acquainted with the terms and conditions involved.

If you choose to leave the sheltered housing bought under these terms you should receive back a proportion of the increased value of the property. The older you are the less you get back. However, this sum will not necessarily be in cash: you may have to satisfy the company of your good health in order to receive a lump sum. Otherwise you receive only an annuity income. It is therefore fair to say that buying under one of these discount schemes could severely limit your options in the future.

You should examine all such schemes very carefully and always obtain independent legal and financial advice.

Getting a special mortgage

If you need to top up your existing capital in order to finance a purchase it may be possible for you to obtain a special 'maturity' mortgage. Many building societies offer these interest-only mortgages to elderly people where the capital is not repaid until the new property is eventually sold. The snag is that you still have to pay the interest each month. People on or near the supplementary benefit level may be able to obtain DHSS assistance with the interest, but otherwise it has to be found from existing income, which may not be easy, particularly when you take into account the fact that the running costs in your new home must also be paid.

Some building societies require you to be at least 60 to qualify for a maturity mortgage but may exercise flexibility on this, particularly where an applicant has already retired.

Selling your home to the council or a housing association

A small number of councils and housing associations may still be able to buy your home from you in return for rehousing you in more suitable accommodation. This practice is not as common as it used to be, mainly because of a lack of smaller properties to offer home owners. If your council or a local housing association can buy your home, you should consult an independent advice centre or a solicitor to check that you are getting a fair price. As you are receiving rented housing in return you will not be offered its full market value.

2·6 Making an outright purchase

Buying ordinary housing

Many older people looking for a house or flat do not particularly wish to buy special housing, and can therefore use the usual sources such as estate agents and newspapers. You can also telephone the **New Homes Marketing Board's Housing Enquiry Service (01 935 7464)**, stating up to three specific areas of preference (not just counties), what type of property you want, the number of bedrooms and your price limit. You will then receive details of any new properties which match your needs.

Think carefully about climbing stairs or living in a hilly area in ten years' time, and the range of questions we list on page 12 will be worth considering.

Buying specially designed housing

Not all of the many builders now developing housing for older people provide sheltered housing (ie with a warden and alarm system). Many are building accommodation with certain special features which make it particularly suitable for older people, but without a warden.

Normally these are freehold bungalows and you should check that they are situated within easy access of shops, public transport and other community facilities. The site and the surrounding area should be fairly flat and not too near noisy factories or busy main roads. Special design features, the number and quality of which vary, may include level or ramped access instead of steps, wider doorways for wheelchairs and walking frames, waist-high sockets and switches, walk-in showers and grab-rails conveniently positioned in the bathroom.

Be wary of housing for older people which is in reality barely distinguishable from conventional housing.

Buying sheltered housing

A large number of developers (and some councils and housing associations) now build sheltered housing for outright sale to older people. Each scheme of flats or bungalows normally has an alarm system and a warden who can keep an unobtrusive eye on residents and arrange for help to be called in an emergency. Once the scheme has been built the developer usually hands over to a separate management organisation (often a housing association), which assumes responsibility for running the scheme.

As this management organisation employs the warden and provides maintenance and other services, it acts as the freeholder. Residents are therefore almost always leaseholders, except in Scotland, where leaseholds do not exist. So as well as having your own rates and bills to pay there will always be a weekly service charge, on average around £7-£14 a week at 1987 prices. Age Concern England has two items of specialist advice on buying sheltered housing: Fact sheet No. 2 *Sheltered Housing for Sale* is available free on receipt of a 9" x 4" SAE from the Information and Policy Department. A booklet entitled *Buyer's Guide to Sheltered Housing* is available at £1 (incl. p + p) from the Marketing Department.

The **Buyer's Guide to Sheltered Housing**, jointly published by Age Concern England and the National Housing and Town Planning Council, looks in detail at the following factors which anyone thinking of buying sheltered housing should consider:

- How experienced are the builder and management organisation?
- How much is the service charge and how big have recent increases been?

- What services does the charge cover?
- Is there a separate 'sinking fund' for major repairs?
- What other one-off or regular charges are there?
- Do you receive back the full amount of its market value when you sell? What deductions are made?
- Can you or your family arrange the sale or does the property have to be re-sold by the management organisation? In either case what administrative charges are made?
- What does the lease say about the procedure if your health deteriorates or you become very frail?
- What exactly is the role of the warden?
- How suitable are the design, location and community facilities?

  The guide does include details of some companies and housing associations selling sheltered housing.

---

*A fuller list of developers is available free on receipt of a 9½" x 6½" SAE from the **New Homes Marketing Board**, 82 New Cavendish Street, London W1M 8AD.*

3·STAYING AT HOME – ADVICE FOR TENANTS

3·1 Council tenants

Responsibility for repairs　You should ensure you are aware which repairs are the council's responsibility and which are yours. Often this is laid down in your tenancy agreement. The council is responsible for the structure and exterior of the property, electrical wiring, water and gas pipes, baths, toilets, basins and sinks. Fixed heaters provided by the council are their responsibility, but not cookers.

A number of small repairs may be your responsibility, as is the internal decoration, although you should check whether the council has any special decorating scheme for elderly people. For example, some councils have a programme of decorating at least one room every three years, providing there is no younger relative living at home.

Getting repair work done　If you are having problems getting repairs done you should contact either your tenants' association (if there is one) or a Citizens Advice Bureau, independent housing advice centre or other local advice centre.

There is a very useful guide entitled **Rights to Repair: A Guide for Council Tenants** *available at £1.95 (incl. p + p) from* **SHAC**, *189a Old Brompton Road, London SW5 0AR.*

When the need for repair work first arises you should contact the housing department or the repairs division, if this is a separate department. Even if you phone them you should also confirm in writing and keep a copy of the letter with the date on it. If the repairs are not carried out after a reasonable period you can ask an environmental health officer from the council to inspect your home and advise the repairs section what work is needed. If you still have no success you may wish to ask a local councillor to take up your complaint. The town hall will have details of your ward councillors.

The 'Right to Repair' Council tenants now have the right to carry out certain minor repairs themselves and claim payment from the council. Only repairs costing between £20 and £200 qualify. To find out more about this rather complicated scheme you should obtain a copy of the leaflet *Right to Repair* (Housing Booklet No. 2) from the council or an advice centre. The scheme has some serious drawbacks and the council may meet only part of the cost of the repair work. You should seek advice from a Citizens Advice Bureau or housing advice centre before carrying out any repairs.

The 'Right to Buy' If you have been a council tenant for at least two years you are entitled to purchase your home from the council under the 'Right to Buy' scheme. For houses the discount varies from 32% after two years' tenancy to 60% after 30 years, with bigger discounts for flats. If you sell within three years of buying, you must repay a proportion of the discount to the council.

If you live in sheltered housing or any other housing which is deemed to be particularly suitable for occupation by elderly people you may not have the right to buy, as it is considered important for councils to be able to maintain their stock of special housing.

You should contact the council if you are interested in this option, but it is worth our pointing out that it can be easy to be tempted into buying your home off the council without fully appreciating the risks involved. We have listed some of the factors worth noting:

- The housing benefit you may now get towards the rent and rates is *not* available for help with mortgage repayments, although you should still continue receiving it towards the rates. (From April 1988 it is likely that all householders will have to pay at least 20% of their rates, whatever their income.)

- As well as the rates you will also have to pay buildings insurance and, if you have bought a flat, there will probably be a service charge too.

- If you are on or near the supplementary benefit level you should think very carefully about whether it would be wise to purchase your home. Although some or all of the interest part of your mortgage repayments can currently be covered by increasing your supplementary pension, this assistance may not be available indefinitely.

- People who have bought their home from the council become responsible for the maintenance of their property. The council will not continue carrying out repairs and you should consider the financial and other implications of this.

The Government leaflet *Your Right to Buy Your Home* is available from councils, housing advice centres and Citizens Advice Bureaux.

If you apply to buy and the council confirms you are eligible, you may find your income is not high enough to obtain the required mortgage. In these circumstances it may be worth asking about the possibility of an interest-only mortgage as described on page 35, but it could be that your income is not really sufficient for any kind of mortgage.

If you have savings which could be put towards the purchase you could enquire about buying your home on a shared ownership basis, as many council tenants have the right to do this. Further details of this scheme are contained in the leaflet *Shared Ownership* (Housing Booklet No. 15) available from councils and advice centres.

3·2 Housing association tenants

If you are a housing association tenant most of the advice given earlier for council tenants applies equally to you, in terms of responsibility for repairs and getting repair work done, although in the first instance you would of course contact your association. The council's environmental health department can order a housing association to carry out repair work.

---

*A useful guide entitled **Rights to Repair: A Guide for Private and Housing Association Tenants** is available at £1.95 (incl. p + p) from **SHAC**, 189a Old Brompton Road, London SW5 0AR.*

If you are a 'secure tenant', as are most housing association tenants, you also have the same rights as council tenants to carry out your own minor repairs and claim payment from the association, under the 'Right to Repair' scheme. As we advised for council tenants, however, if you are having problems getting repairs done you should contact your tenants' association (if there is one) or a local advice centre.

If you are the tenant of a charitable housing association you do not have the right to buy your home but you may be entitled to apply to the association for financial assistance to enable you to make a purchase in the private market. If you are interested you should ask your association about these 'transferable discounts'. Details of this scheme are contained in the Housing Corporation's leaflet *Home Ownership for Tenants of Charitable Housing Associations*, available from your housing association or an advice centre.

3·3 Private tenants

For tenants who rent from a private landlord, getting repair work carried out can be especially difficult. If you have a written tenancy agreement you should check which repairs are your responsibility and which are the landlord's. Even if you do not have a written agreement, in most cases if you have become a tenant after 1961, the landlord will still be responsible for most repairs under the 1985 Landlord and Tenant Act. If you have been a tenant in the same property since before 1961 the situation may not be so clear and you should seek advice.

If you cannot get your landlord to carry out repairs for which he is responsible you can ask the local council's environmental health department to take action, and it will hopefully not be necessary for you to have to take court action yourself.

The **SHAC** booklet mentioned in the preceding section contains very useful guidance for private tenants.

It must be stressed that if you are experiencing any kind of problem in a privately rented property, you should avoid signing any documents sent or given to you and instead seek advice from a solicitor, Citizens Advice Bureau, law centre, or housing advice centre.

*Shelter's regional housing aid centres have considerable experience of landlord/tenant problems and you can get the address of your nearest centre from **Shelter**, 88 Old Street, London EC1V 9AX. Tel: 01 253 0202.*

Improvements to the property Getting improvements done to the home can also be notoriously difficult for private tenants, but if you wish to carry out improvements which the landlord is not intending to do himself, he cannot withhold his consent without good reason, if you are a fully protected tenant. Many private tenants are entitled to apply for an improvement grant, as described on page 50, although grants do not cover the whole cost of the work and you will need to seek advice about raising the finance for the remainder.

Unfortunately we are not able to give detailed advice here on tackling repairs problems, or on such matters as disputes over the rent, harassment, being threatened with eviction etc., but if you are having difficulties you should contact a local housing advice centre, Citizens Advice Bureau, law centre or similar advice centre.

Buying as a sitting tenant Some elderly private tenants find themselves in a situation where their landlord is offering to sell them the house or flat as the sitting tenant. Always seek professional advice as the pros and cons of buying from your landlord need careful consideration.

- The obvious advantage is that as a sitting tenant you will be paying less than the property's actual market value when vacant. But do obtain an independent valuation and don't be afraid to barter over the price.

- Getting repairs will not necessarily be any easier after you have purchased the property. If you have bought a freehold property your ability to get repairs done will be mainly dependent on whether you can finance the work. If you have bought a leasehold flat without also buying the freehold or a share in the freehold, then the freeholder will still be responsible for arranging structural repairs.

- You can find yourself in deep water if, after you have bought the property, the freeholder undertakes extensive repair or improvement work. As a leaseholder you will be responsible for paying for your share of the work's cost. An unscrupulous landlord may even delay carrying out repairs until you have bought the leasehold.

- There is a risk that you may be tempted into buying from the landlord when the property is not really suitable for your needs, especially if the landlord is pressurising you to make a decision.

4·STAYING AT HOME - ADVICE FOR HOME OWNERS

4·1 Help with minor repairs, decorating and gardening

Getting help is not always easy, but in some areas there are schemes which arrange for minor repairs, decorating and gardening jobs to be carried out by volunteers or people working on Manpower Services Commission schemes. If there is no special housing agency service in your area (see page 47) you should ask your local Age Concern group, Council for Voluntary Service, Citizens Advice Bureau or social services department if they run (or know of) any scheme.

4·2 Bigger repairs and improvements - identifying the need

You may have no doubts as to what work needs doing to your home, but many older people either lack sufficient knowledge of house maintenance or are reluctant to admit there may be faults which need remedying. Anxieties about finding a reliable builder, fear of the disruption which might be caused and an inability to pay are other common reasons why repair work is not carried out. Nevertheless you should consider a number of questions, such as:

- Is there dampness or rotten wood anywhere?
- Can you tell how sound the roof is?
- Are the heating and insulation good enough to enable you to get through cold weather in comfort?
- Are the kitchen, bathroom and toilet facilities safe and easy to use?
- How convenient is the layout of your home? Would it be easier having a downstairs bathroom?

If you don't feel there is a need for any immediate improvements, it is worth looking ahead a few years. As well as looking at the layout to assess whether it will be convenient in the future, you might consider whether it would be helpful to have grab-rails by the bath and toilet or even a shower instead of a bath. Putting lever handles on taps for easier turning, or raising electric sockets to make them easier to reach, are other examples.

A booklet published by Age Concern England and the National Housing and Town Planning Council, entitled *Are you Living Comfortably?* is available at £1.50 (incl. p + p) from Age Concern England's Marketing Department.

The booklet contains more detailed advice about making your home easier to live in, and highlights the value of having your home professionally surveyed in order to identify any necessary repair work. It includes a checklist of different parts of the property which may need looking at:

Externally
External decorations; Rainwater pipes and gutters; Roof finishes and fixtures; External walls; Drains; Paths and steps; Doors and door frames; Windows and window frames.

Internally
Heating and insulation installations; Electrical wiring and fixtures; Service pipes and plumbing; Waste pipes and soil stack; Sanitary fittings; Internal walls and decorations; Floors and floor coverings.

4·3 Seeking specialist advice on repairs

Housing agency services

In a small but increasing number of areas there are special agency advice schemes which help people to arrange repairs and improvements to their home. These schemes have various titles such as 'Staying Put' or 'Care and Repair' projects and are run by voluntary organisations, housing associations and local authorities. Most are aimed specifically at older people.

These schemes do not actually fund the repair work but once they have arranged for an initial survey to be carried out and plans to be drawn up, they will help you through the often complex procedures of applying for a council grant (if available) and/or building society loan. Where appropriate they will liaise with the DHSS on your behalf and will also appoint builders and keep an eye on the work's progress. All these agency schemes are non profit-making but may charge a fee to cover staff and other costs, in which case this can normally be included in the grant or loan.

Some local councils which do not run a full agency service may still be able to provide advice, particularly on the technical (ie building) side, to elderly people who are applying for a grant. They may also be able to help you arrange finance for the part of the work not covered by the grant. Any fee will normally be included in the grant.

Your local Age Concern group, council housing or environmental health department should be able to tell you if there is a special housing agency service in your area.

Other sources of advice

If there is no special agency service in your area, getting good professional advice about repairs and improvements and then finding a reliable builder is not always easy, but there are a few pointers worth following:

Finding a surveyor If you have applied for a home

improvement grant from the council or for a building society loan, then some councils and building societies will arrange the survey. If you are not receiving help from either of these sources, the council's environmental health department may be able to recommend local surveyors.

A local housing association may be able to arrange for their surveyor to visit you, although they are normally very busy. Some voluntary organisations may have access to a surveyor, so ask at your local Age Concern group or Council for Voluntary Service. You can ask the local Citizens Advice Bureau about the **Chartered Surveyors Voluntary Service**, which aims to help people who are uncertain how to obtain professional advice. The CAB should be able to tell you whether a surveyor can help you and whether you are eligible for help free of charge.

Before any surveyor inspects your property you should ask what the fee will be. You will still have to pay this even if no subsequent repair work is carried out. Otherwise the fee is likely to be a percentage (say 10% or 15%) of the cost of the work, but higher if the surveyor takes over the whole process of arranging the work and the financing of it (only a few surveyors will do this).

Finding a builder There are *no* easy ways of finding a reliable builder. The local council's environmental health department may be able to recommend local builders although they will not be able to guarantee or be responsible for their reliability. Personal recommendation from friends or neighbours is useful for small building jobs. But for large-scale work, it is advisable to use a builder who is backed by a reputable guarantee scheme.

The two main schemes are run by the **Building Employers Confederation** and the **Federation of Master Builders**. For a charge of 1% of the cost of the work, it is guaranteed not only that the work will be fully completed as agreed but also that any faults arising later will be rectified by another builder.

*Information on how these schemes operate and details of builders registered under either scheme can be obtained from: **The B.E.C. Building Trust Ltd.**, Medway House, London Road, Maidstone,*

*Kent ME16 8JH and **The Federation of Master Builders**, Gordon
Fisher House, 33 John Street, London WC1N 2BB.*

**You should always obtain at least two or three estimates from
different builders before making your final choice.**

Sources of advice for people with disabilities

If you are becoming more frail or suffer from a particular
disability and need advice about making your home more easy
to manage, you can contact the social services department to
arrange for an occupational therapist (O.T.) to visit and make
recommendations. O.T.'s assess how particular disabilities
affect your capacity to get around and carry out household
tasks and they can suggest adaptations to alleviate the
difficulties. If improvement grant work is subsequently
carried out, the O.T. should ensure that her recommendations
are followed by the surveyor and builder. Unfortunately
O.T.'s are generally very busy as most of them work in
understaffed departments, so you may have to wait some
months before you receive a visit.

Where major adaptation work is being carried out, you will
need to employ an architect, whether or not you are getting
home improvement grant assistance with the work. The O.T.
should see the plans drawn up, particularly if the architect
does not have much experience of designing for people with
disabilities. The **Centre on Environment for the Handicapped**
runs the **Architectural Advisory Service**, which maintains a
register of architects and other professionals with experience
of designing for elderly and disabled people, including major
house adaptation work.

*Information on this service can be obtained from **Centre on
Environment for the Handicapped**, 35 Great Smith Street, London
SW1P 3BJ. Tel: 01 222 7980.*

4·4 Financial help with repairs and improvements

Assuming you have no substantial income or savings of your own, there are two main ways in which it may be possible to obtain financial assistance with larger repair work – a home improvement grant from the council or a special loan from a building society.

Home improvement grants

Local councils can give grants which cover a proportion of the cost of certain types of repair and improvement work. Although the grants system has been under review for almost two years now, at the time of writing (April 1987) it is still the age, rateable value and overall condition of the property, rather than the needs and wishes of the occupant, which govern whether a grant can be given. For example, even if you only want a particular improvement such as rewiring or the installation of central heating, it is normally necessary for the council to insist on a package of further repairs or improvements, whether or not you want them.

Furthermore, major cuts in the amount of money allocated by the Government to local councils for spending on housing mean that in many areas grants are very difficult to obtain, and there may be a long waiting list. It may sometimes be that only intermediate grants, for the provision of basic amenities, can be obtained, as these are mandatory (ie the council has to give them). A number of councils, however, give priority to applications from elderly and disabled people.

The different types of grant available are explained in detail in the leaflet *Home Improvement Grants* (Housing Booklet No. 14) available from the council or advice centres, but briefly the three main types of grant are as follows:

Intermediate grants These are mandatory, so if your home has no inside toilet, bath, hot and cold water supply or any other basic amenity (but not including central heating) the council must give a grant towards the cost of providing them and carrying out any associated repair work. To qualify, the house or flat must have been built or converted before 1961.

Improvement grants   These are discretionary, which means the council can decide whether or not to give them. They are available towards the cost of major improvements (and any associated repair work) required to raise the standard of any property built before 1961, providing the rateable value does not exceed £225, or £400 in Greater London. If you live in a Housing Action Area or if you are disabled these rateable value limits do not apply. A wide range of work can be covered by improvement grants but the installation of central heating, and other one-off improvements, are covered only if they are part of a larger programme of work.

Repair grants   These too are only discretionary, and are available towards the cost of major structural repairs to properties built before 1919. Unfortunately inter-war houses and flats do not therefore qualify, even though many are in need of repair. The replacement of worn fixtures (such as baths) is not covered, nor is routine maintenance work, in which category electrical rewiring is included. As with central heating, rewiring *can* be grant-aided if it is part of a larger programme of work being carried out. The property's rateable value must not exceed £225, or £400 in Greater London.

How much will the grant be?   For each type of grant there is an 'eligible expense limit', ie a maximum sum that can be covered by the grant, and the grant will only meet a certain percentage of this sum. This varies from 50% to 90% depending on the type of grant, the location and condition of the property and on your own circumstances. For example, in some cases where the council decides that you would not be able to pay for your share of the work without undue hardship, you may be given a 90% grant.

Full details of the eligible expense limits and grant rules are set out in the leaflet *Home Improvement Grants* (Housing Booklet No. 14), mentioned earlier in this section, but in order to give you an indication, the following table shows the maximum sum that can be covered by a grant. The figures are correct as at April 1987 and have not been increased since April 1983.

Remember that the actual grant you receive will only be a percentage of these limits

	Outside London	Greater London
Intermediate grant	£ 2,275	£ 3,005
Repairs accompanying Intermediate grant work	£ 3,000	£ 4,200
Repairs grant	£ 4,800	£ 6,600
Improvement grants:		
* priority	£ 10,200	£ 13,800
non-priority	£ 6,600	£ 9,000

* A priority case for an improvement grant is a house which is lacking standard amenities, is in need of substantial and structural repair, is in a Housing Action Area, or is being adapted for a disabled person.

The council will tell you which category of grant the work you require comes under, and whether yours is a priority case. If you cannot meet the remaining cost of the work from your own savings you will probably need to consider applying for a special interest-only loan from a building society (see later in this section).

Scotland   There are some different rules relating to the grants system in Scotland. The main points are as follows:

• There are no intermediate grants in Scotland. The equivalent is an improvement grant for providing standard amenities.

• Both repairs and improvement grants can be given for properties built before 15 June 1964.

• There are different rateable value limits in Scotland, varying from district to district.

• Some eligible expense limits are also different in Scotland.

Special help for people with disabilities   Over and above the normal grants system there are certain special conditions aimed at helping people with disabilities, who are normally given priority when applying for assistance:

- Mandatory intermediate grants are available to provide extra standard amenities if the existing ones cannot be reached by a disabled occupant.

- Improvement grants are available to adapt a house or flat for a disabled person, and various types of adaptation work are covered, such as putting in a downstairs bedroom or bathroom, installing a stairlift, or providing ramps for people who use wheelchairs. Appropriate bathroom and kitchen alterations are also covered, as is electrical work to put switches and sockets at more convenient heights instead of at skirting board level.

- Both intermediate and improvement grants for disabled people qualify for higher eligible expense limits and grant rates, and the property need not have been built before 1961. Also, rateable value limits do not apply.

Generally a grant will be given only if an occupational therapist confirms that the work is required: thus any grant application will involve the social services department as well as the housing/environmental health department.

Under the 1970 Chronically Sick and Disabled Persons Act social services departments have a duty to assist in making arrangements for necessary adaptations. This includes the provision of both financial assistance and help with assessing what work is needed, by having plans prepared and liaising with other council departments. Social services departments also have a duty to help with any necessary adaptation work not covered by home improvement grants, and with the provision of any additional facilities which will make the property safer, more comfortable and more convenient. There is considerable variation amongst authorities in giving assistance under this Act.

*If you are having difficulties getting help, one organisation which might be able to advise you is **RADAR**, The Royal Association for Disability and Rehabilitation, 25 Mortimer Street, London W1N 8AB. Tel: 01 637 5400.*

Applying for a grant   If you wish to apply for a grant and there is no special agency service in your area you should contact the improvement grants section of your council, normally in the environmental health or housing department. You should *never* make any arrangements to start work before getting the go-ahead from the council, as you will lose all entitlement to grant assistance.

Insulation grants

These are available towards the cost of insulating lofts and lagging hot water tanks and pipes. The lagging of cold water tanks situated in the loft also qualifies. If you receive supplementary benefit or housing benefit (ie rent or rate rebate) you can claim a grant of up to 90% of the cost of materials, up to a maximum of £95. Elderly people who do not receive supplementary or housing benefit cannot obtain an insulation grant.

You should ask the grants section of your local council whether you qualify for a grant. You will not qualify if you begin the work without obtaining the council's approval. A leaflet entitled *Save Money on Loft Insulation* can be obtained from council offices and advice centres.

Interest-only loans (maturity loans)

Where there are no grants available, or where you still need additional money to top up the grant, it is becoming increasingly common to look into the possibility of getting an interest-only maturity loan. Some councils still make these loans available but they are now usually obtained from a building society. Although your first reaction may be reluctance to start borrowing in your later years, these loans are in fact specifically aimed at older people, and are given on special terms.

Supposing you need £3,000 to replace the roof, and no grant assistance is available, you could consider applying for an interest-only loan, which is not repaid until the property is eventually sold. As you pay the interest due each month, only the original £3,000 you borrowed is taken out of the proceeds of the sale, even if that is in many years' time. If you have children you will probably want to discuss this with them, but neither you nor your family need worry about an interest-only loan seriously decreasing the assets you pass on when you die. In most areas of the country repair work will either protect or increase the property's value, as well as make your home more comfortable, and probably safer.

Having to pay the interest each month is often the problem with these loans. Interest rates at April 1987 mean that the repayments on a £3,000 interest-only loan would be around £5 per week (ie around £22 per month). Interest rates can of course fluctuate and you should always check how much the repayments will be.

If you receive supplementary benefit, or if the interest payments would take you below the supplementary benefit scale rate, you should be entitled to assistance from the DHSS, who will increase your benefit to cover some or all of the interest payments, subject to two particular conditions:

- The repair work involved must be classified as major repairs necessary to maintain the fabric of the house or improve its 'fitness for occupation'.
- For the payments to be met in full by the DHSS your savings must not exceed £500. If you do have more than £500 the DHSS expects you to use the surplus to pay for as much of the work as possible before it meets the interest on what is left. For example, if you have £800 savings but do not wish to use any of it, the DHSS will only pay interest on £2,700 of a £3,000 loan, as your savings are £300 over the permissible £500.

Home owners who are not entitled to supplementary benefit assistance, yet who cannot pay the interest from their limited income, often ask whether the interest can be allowed to 'roll up', and not be repaid until the capital itself is repaid when the property is eventually sold. Many building societies are reluctant to permit this, but it may be possible in certain cases for some of the interest to be rolled up. The problem is that by doing this the amount of capital that must eventually be repaid can increase substantially, mainly because no tax relief is given on interest which is rolled up.

Other points to note about interest-only loans include:

- There will be a building society valuation fee and some other charges, but these can normally be included in the loan itself.

- Building societies are generally reluctant to give interest-only loans for minor repair work, as they would still have to charge the necessary fees for administering the loan. On a small job the fees could therefore be high, in proportion to the size of the loan. As a rough indication you may find some societies unwilling to lend less than around £1,000 at 1987 prices.

- If you have a mortgage already and if the lender will allow it, it is well worth keeping a small amount outstanding, even as little as £1. You may be looking forward to paying off your mortgage and claiming the deeds, but if you leave this small amount unpaid, it should be easier and cheaper to arrange to increase the mortgage rather than take out a completely new loan in order to pay for repairs and improvements in the future. Also it will mean that the deeds are safely looked after.

- The minimum age limit to qualify for a maturity loan varies, but is often around 60. Flexibility may be exercised though, especially where an applicant is already retired.

- Not all building societies give maturity loans and some restrict them to existing account holders.

You may wish to check with your local council's finance department to see if they give interest-only loans, but if not, you should shop around local building societies.

Conventional loans

Some building societies and banks will consider giving older people a normal repayment loan, probably payable over a period such as 10 or 15 years, but as both capital and interest are being repaid the monthly repayments will be higher than in the case of an interest-only loan.

If the loan is for major repairs or essential improvements, people on or near the supplementary benefit level would still be eligible for DHSS assistance with the interest element of the repayments, but no help is available to repay the capital.

As was said earlier, it is likely to be easier and cheaper for you to obtain a loan if, instead of paying off the mortgage, you keep your account open by leaving a nominal amount unpaid.

Not all repairs and home improvements are eligible for tax relief, so check this with your lender.

Paying for smaller repair work

Unfortunately it is often very difficult to obtain any financial assistance for smaller repair work. Not only is such work not normally covered by home improvement grants or maturity loans but there are few other sources to turn to if, for example, you need £500-£1,000 for rewiring. It is not impossible to obtain a maturity loan for this amount, but the fees will be high in proportion to the size of the loan. Building societies may ask you to consider getting other repair work done, to increase the loan to around £1,000 or more.

Unsecured loans   The new Building Societies Act, which came into force at the beginning of 1987, gives societies the power to make available unsecured loans for relatively small amounts. (Previously, even if your home was clearly worth many thousands of pounds and you only required a very small loan, building societies were required by law to mortgage the property. This was time-consuming and expensive.)

An unsecured loan is easier to arrange but the interest rate is normally higher than for a mortgage. Not all building societies make unsecured loans available and terms can vary with those that do. You should therefore enquire at local building society branches to see if you can obtain an unsecured loan and, if so, how much it will cost compared to a normal loan or mortgage.

Bank loans   These are not cheap, but if you think you might be able to afford the repayments you should make enquiries, particularly if you have an account already.

Finance companies   Any companies other than building societies and banks which offer loans to older people should be avoided. Many are unscrupulous and charge very high interest rates.

DHSS single payments   Until April 1988, if you receive supplementary benefit and have savings of £500 or less, you may be able to obtain a 'single payment', which is a grant from the DHSS, for essential repairs and any resulting decoration which is necessary. The total cost must not exceed £325 and you must get the approval of your local social security office before starting any of the work. The cost of simple draught-proofing and essential decorations can also be covered by DHSS single payments, as can the cost of survey fees incurred when you apply for a building society or bank loan, if the fees are not included in the loan. Legal fees cannot be covered by single payments.

Single payments are becoming increasingly difficult to obtain, due to Government cutbacks, and none will be available from April 1988, when the whole social security system changes. Under the new system, the only help available towards repairs will be in the form of a loan from the 'Social Fund', if the local DHSS approves. The loan must be repaid by deductions from your weekly benefit.

From April 1988 you should ask about the new system at a welfare rights advice centre or Citizens Advice Bureau, and full details will be contained in Age Concern England's annual booklet *Your Rights* at that time.

Weekly addition for insurance and minor repairs If you already receive a supplementary pension you should ensure that it includes a weekly addition (£1.85 as at April 1987) towards the cost of minor repairs and house insurance. This addition will not be available after April 1988. In the meantime you can ask your local social security office for Form A124 which shows exactly how your supplementary pension has been worked out, and what has been included in it.

Age Concern England offers two separate insurance policies, one for household contents and one for buildings. Write for details to the Insurance Department, enclosing a large SAE.

Charitable trusts In a few areas there may be a charity or trust fund which can help towards the cost of smaller repair work. Your local Age Concern group or Council for Voluntary Service may know of any such local charities or trusts, but this will only occasionally be a likely source of assistance.

4·5 Raising an income from your home

Many older people are in the frustrating position of having a low income, yet owning a property, with their capital therefore tied up in bricks and mortar. If you are a single person aged at least 70, or a couple with combined ages of at least 150, you may wish to consider using all or part of the capital value of your home to raise either an annuity income or a lump sum, whilst continuing to live in the house.

To the great disappointment of many older people who have not yet reached these qualifying ages, there are currently no other means of unlocking capital tied up in the home, whatever its value. There are one or two companies with lower minimum age requirements but the income or lump sum they offer will for most people not be worth seriously considering.

For those people who do qualify, the two main ways of using the capital tied up in a property are through home income plans and home reversion schemes.

Home income plans

A home income plan, sometimes called a mortgage annuity scheme, is the more common of the two types of scheme for raising money from your home. It involves using a proportion of the property's value, say 70%, to obtain an interest-only loan, which is not repaid until the home is eventually sold. The loan is used to buy an annuity (ie a lifetime income). Part of the annuity income must be used to pay the interest on the loan, but the remainder is your net income to spend as you wish. Tax relief is normally available on the loan interest you pay.

The proportion of the property's value which can be used for a home income plan varies from scheme to scheme, but is normally between 65% and 80%, up to a maximum of £30,000. To take an example, if your house is worth £40,000 you could with some schemes obtain a loan of up to £30,000 with which an annuity income would be obtained. If the property were to be sold in 10 years' time for £55,000 the £30,000 loan would be repaid and the remaining £25,000 would still belong to you or your estate.

Annuities are calculated on the basis of average life expectancies, so the older you are the bigger the annuity income will be, and single people receive more than couples. Also a single man, who has a shorter average life expectancy will receive more than a woman of a similar age.

With most schemes, you can if you wish start off with an initial cash sum, in return for the subsequent annuity income being reduced. For example, with a £30,000 loan you should be able to receive an initial sum of around £2,400. Another option normally available is whether or not to protect your loan. If you choose to obtain 'capital protection' this will mean that should you die during the three years after taking out the loan your estate will receive back a proportion of the loan: 75% during the first year, 50% during the second year and 25% during the third year. If you opt for capital protection the annuity income itself will be slightly reduced.

Some other important points worth noting:

- If you currently receive either supplementary benefit or housing benefit (formerly rates rebate), the extra income or capital from one of these schemes will seriously affect your entitlement to such benefits, which you could lose altogether. It is likely that the extra income or capital would need to be fairly substantial if it is to compensate for the loss of benefit, and you should look into this very carefully.

- Taking up a home income plan in order to provide finance for repair or improvement work should not be done without first looking into whether there are any other less drastic means of funding the work. Consult the earlier section on help with repairs and improvements.

- You should obtain quotes from more than one company, as the income can vary considerably, depending on various factors, such as which annuity the company selects and what its interest rate is.

- Some schemes have fixed interest rates and others variable. In the case of a home income plan with a variable interest rate, you should note that if the interest rate rises your income will decrease. Likewise if the rate falls, your income will increase. You may feel it is safer to select a scheme with a fixed interest rate.

- Taking up a home income plan does not mean you cannot move in the future, but you should check exactly what the procedure would be for transferring the loan and annuity to another property. Inevitably, if you have a home income plan, moving home in the future will be more complicated.
- You should never commit yourself to any scheme before seeking independent, professional legal and financial advice, and if you have children or other close relatives you will probably want to discuss it with them too.

Home reversion schemes

Another less common way of raising money from your property is through a home reversion scheme, which involves actually selling the home to a reversions company, normally for a one-off lump sum, although one or two schemes provide an annuity income. You stay living in your home, paying a nominal rent such as £1 per month, but it is important to note that responsibility for maintenance is still yours, not the company's.

On your death, or on the death of both partners in the case of a couple, the entire value of the property passes to the company, so it would be an option to consider if you do not need or wish to pass on any part of the value to children or other relatives or friends. Hopefully if you have children they will urge you to make use of the property's capital if you wish.

Much of the information given above on home income plans applies equally to reversion schemes, so the size of the lump sum you would receive through a reversion scheme is dependent on your age, sex and whether you are single or a couple. In many cases the cash sum received will be substantially less than half the property's current market value, so you would want to think extremely carefully before committing yourself, and the need to seek independent, professional legal and financial advice is particularly crucial.

Information on raising an income

Fact sheet No. 12 *Raising an Income from your Home* is available free on receipt of a 9" x 4" SAE from Age Concern England's Information and Policy Department. It includes brief details of those schemes known to Age Concern, but inclusion does not constitute a recommendation, and Age Concern cannot advise on which company is the best, as this very much depends on your individual circumstances.

A detailed booklet entitled *Using Your Home as Capital* can be obtained from Age Concern England's Marketing Department after October 1987. Please check the price before ordering.

4·6 Letting your home

This section applies to council and private tenants, as well as to home owners.

This is an option considered by a number of elderly people, particularly home owners, but even if you have a large property you should think very carefully about letting a room or taking in lodgers. Do consider whether you might find it difficult sharing the house if you are not used to doing so.

Being a landlord or landlady can be quite a complex matter. For very good reasons, many tenants are now fairly well protected and you need to ensure you do not get into a situation where you cannot regain possession of the whole of your house, should you decide you no longer wish to let out part of it. This should not be difficult, as the 1980 Housing Act introduced new rules to make it simpler for resident landlords to let rooms in their home by means of a 'restricted contract'.

If the landlord and tenant live in the same house, and if a rent is charged and no meals provided, any letting made on or after 28th November 1980 will be a restricted contract. If you made a letting before this it may still count as a restricted contract, but special rules apply and you should check the situation with an advice centre. No formalities nor any written agreement are required for letting under a restricted contract, although it is of course necessary for the landlord and tenant to agree the rent.

Both the landlord and tenant can if they wish apply to the local rent tribunal at any time for a 'reasonable rent' to be registered. All reasonable rents are shown on a register which can be examined at the local rent assessment panel office. Your local Citizens Advice Bureau will give you the address of the rent tribunal and panel offices for your area.

A tenant with a restricted contract does not have full security of tenure but the landlord must follow certain procedures before the tenant can be made to leave. Details of these procedures and further information about lettings are set out in the leaflet *Letting Rooms in Your Home* (Housing Booklet No. 4), available from advice centres.

If you are considering letting out part of your home, or if you have already done so and are experiencing problems, it is vital that you seek advice from a solicitor, Citizens Advice Bureau, law centre or housing advice centre. The same applies if you wish to let a home you have bought for later on in your retirement but which you are not yet occupying, in which case the leaflet you should obtain is *Letting Your Home or Retirement Home* (Housing Booklet No. 5).

You must remember that rental income from tenants will affect any supplementary benefit or housing benefit you receive.

4·7 Donating your home to a charity

We know of only one charity to which you can donate your home while continuing to live there, with the responsibility for rates, insurance and external maintenance of the property passing to the charity. This is Help the Aged, *not* Age Concern. If you are interested in this option you should contact them at the address below, and they will arrange for a surveyor to visit. You would of course use a solicitor for such a transaction and you should check very carefully on what arrangements will be made for repairs to be carried out if and when they become necessary:

Information about this scheme can be obtained from **Help the Aged Housing Division**, *1 Ward Street, Guildford GU3 4LH. Tel: 0483 571772.*

5·SUPPORT, SECURITY AND COMFORT AT HOME

The purpose of this section is to give brief advice on certain matters affecting elderly people who wish to stay at home, whether they are owners or tenants.

5·1 Support services at home

An important factor for some elderly people wishing to remain at home rather than move is the availability of assistance with domestic or personal tasks, from social services or other sources. It is pointless for you to move reluctantly if the support you need can be provided at home, and for many people who have tried without success to move, it becomes imperative to look into what help could be obtained.

It is possible to give only a general indication as to what sort of help might be available. The public spending restrictions of recent years have meant that in most areas there are insufficient support services to meet demand, and in any case provision varies greatly between areas. You should discuss your needs with the doctor, or social worker and relatives, where appropriate. The social worker in particular should know about what services are run locally, but you can also consult your local Age Concern group, Council for Voluntary Service or Citizens Advice Bureau.

Services such as home help assistance, meals on wheels or day-care are available in most areas, but the quality of these services, the charges for them and the extent to which they are available varies considerably. Other services operated in some areas include hospital after-care schemes to assist people who have recently left hospital, chiropody services, voluntary transport schemes and services to support people who care for elderly relatives. There may also be gardening and decorating schemes.

Some voluntary agencies (including a number of local Age Concern groups) provide domiciliary services such as attendant schemes which recruit carers who are a cross between a home help and a good neighbour. Such carers might be able to offer a flexible service providing care at unusual times such as early in the morning and late at night.

If you need nursing care or help with personal tasks such as bathing and dressing, you should ask your doctor whether arrangements can be made for a community/district nurse to visit you regularly. Voluntary agencies such as the local branch of the British Red Cross Society may also be able to offer help.

Finding 'companions' or living-in help can be a solution and sources worth consulting are listed in Age Concern England's fact sheet No. 6 *Companions and Living-in Help* available free on receipt of a 9" x 4" SAE from the Information and Policy Department.

There may be local agencies in your area who recruit staff to work on an hourly or daily basis and there can sometimes be financial assistance towards this. Anyone entitled to receive supplementary pension can claim a Domestic Assistance Addition to cover the cost of employing a domestic helper if they, and all others in their household, are unable to cook and clean for themselves because of ill health, infirmity, disability or heavy family responsibilities.

The following checklist is intended as a brief guide to what services might be available locally, which organisation provides them and how to go about contacting them:

Adaptations to the home council's housing or environmental health department; social services (for occupational therapist)

Aids/specialist equipment for daily living social services; district health authority; British Red Cross Society

Alarm systems council's housing or social services department; private firms

Carers' groups such as Crossroads Care Schemes social services; voluntary organisations

Chiropody district health authority; private chiropodists

Day centres and day care social services; voluntary organisations such as Age Concern

Day hospitals district health authority

District nurse district nursing service (through G.P.)

Health visitor through G.P. or health centre

Home help social services

Incontinence service district nursing service (through G.P.)

Library services including mobile libraries for housebound people council's libraries department

Lunch clubs social services; voluntary organisations such as Age Concern or WRVS

Meals on wheels social services; voluntary organisations such as WRVS

Nail-cutting services district health authority

Night nursing district nursing service (through G.P.)

Occupational therapy social services; district health authority via hospital

Physiotherapy district health authority via hospital

Short-stay residential care social services; private and voluntary homes

Sitting service to give carers a break social services; voluntary organisations

Social clubs social services; voluntary organisations such as Age Concern

Stroke clubs social services; district health authority via hospital; voluntary organisations

Speech therapy district health authority

Social workers social services

Visiting schemes voluntary organisations such as Age Concern

5·2 Specialist aids to everyday living

Although some elderly people could well benefit from having structural adaptations made to their home (see page 53), there are simpler ways to make life around the house easier to cope with, and safer too. As you get more frail and unsteady on your feet, simple tasks like getting dressed, taking a bath and going to the lavatory can all become more difficult.

Advice and information If you are having difficulty in coping you can ask the council's social services department for an occupational therapist (O.T.) to visit you. O.T.'s advise on fixtures, fittings and equipment which can range from walking frames to safety grab-rails, bath seats and commodes as well as kitchen utensils to make the preparation and cooking of food easier for people with arthritic hands.

The Information Service of the **Disabled Living Foundation** can supply details of specialist equipment, including stockists, as well as a list of addresses of regional aids centres where you can go and see the permanent exhibition yourself, usually by appointment.

Many useful items are readily available in high street stores. Some larger branches of Boots stock a selection of aids and all branches should be able to give you a copy of their booklet *Personal Independence* from which you can order items.

Further advice on aids and adaptations is included in the booklet *Are you Living Comfortably?* mentioned on page 46.

5·3 Telephones

If you do not have a telephone you may wish to consider the advantages of having one installed, such as being able to ring for the doctor or other help in an emergency. Either now or in the future you may find you tend not to go out as often and a telephone could ensure you still keep in touch with friends.

Fact sheet No. 28 *Telephone Costs – Sources of Financial Help*, describing the assistance which may be available to some elderly people with the cost of installing and using a telephone, is available free on receipt of a 9" x 4" SAE from the Information and Policy Department of Age Concern England.

5·4 Personal alarm systems

You will probably have noticed the recent increase in the number of companies advertising personal alarm systems for elderly people to use in the event of an emergency. There has also been a large increase in the number of local authorities (along with a few housing associations) installing alarms in the homes of elderly tenants, and in some cases owner-occupiers.

Although such systems are in no way a replacement for human contact they can offer some security and peace of mind to elderly people living alone, often feeling isolated and vulnerable. It may sometimes be your relatives who are seeking peace of mind and you may want to be reassured that just because you have an emergency alarm system you do not receive fewer visits from friends, relatives or social services! As interest in alarm systems is clearly increasing some guidelines may be useful, if only for possible future use.

Personal alarms enable elderly people to summon help in an emergency by pressing a button or pulling a cord to send a signal to the special unit attached to the telephone. The alarm is activated either by a hanging cord or by a portable trigger, which in most cases can be worn round the neck like a pendant, over the wrist or hand-held. Two-way speech systems enable you to speak to the person answering your call, even if you are some way from the telephone, although the range and quality of the sound varies considerably between systems.

With most systems, when the telephone is activated it rings whatever telephone numbers it has been programmed to dial. It may be the mobile warden, relatives or friends living nearby, or the control centre, who will summon appropriate emergency services if necessary. If the first telephone number produces no response the second should automatically be called, and so on until contact is made. It is very important that any alarm system is linked into a control centre which is staffed 24 hours a day.

If you are interested in obtaining a personal alarm you should first check whether the housing or social services department of your local council runs an alarm system for people in their own homes. A fair number of councils do this, but rules vary as to who is eligible. However, even if you do not qualify it may be possible for you to buy your own alarm and have it connected to the council's control centre. Some councils run a mobile warden service to answer emergency alarm calls but you should always check exactly what the arrangements are for answering calls.

If you do choose to buy a personal alarm privately a number of points are worth watching out for. A report in the Consumer Association's WHICH? Magazine in July 1986 (available in larger public libraries) following a major survey by the Research Institute for Consumer Affairs, found a number of faults in several alarm systems and advised prospective purchasers to consider certain factors, including the following:

- You should not buy any system which does not have a control centre, nor any which fails to work during a power-cut.
- You should only consider systems which make several attempts to get through, and which enable the alarm to be set off again shortly after the first call. It should also be possible to cancel a false alarm.

- You should make it a condition of purchase that the trigger range is tested from various points around your home and garden.
- The purchase price of an alarm system does not normally include the use of the control centre or repairs and maintenance, which must be paid for through annual charges.

*Information on alarm systems available for purchase is available from the Information Service of the **Disabled Living Foundation**, 380-384 Harrow Road, London W9 2HU. Tel: 01 289 6111.*

5·5 Home security

There is a section on home security in the booklet *Are you Living Comfortably?* (see page 46), but a few important points are worth highlighting here.

Every police station has a Crime Prevention Officer (CPO) who can visit your home and advise on how you can make it more secure. CPO's can advise on different types of doors, windows and locks, the quality of which is of prime importance in keeping a home secure. CPO's are normally very busy but you should try and take advantage of this service and contact your local police station. A CPO can also advise on whether there is a local Neighbourhood Watch Scheme already in existence or proposed for the future.

Some local councils and welfare organisations such as Age Concern groups produce booklets advising on security and crime prevention, and may be able to tell you whether there are any local Manpower Services Commission schemes which fit locks and security fittings for the cost of materials only.

They may also have a grant scheme to help people finance certain security measures, although there is no help of this kind available on a national scale unless the security work is part of a larger programme of work being financed by a home improvement grant from the council. You should also check with your local Age Concern group to see if they know of any charitable trust which could be approached for financial assistance, although in many areas this kind of help will not be available.

5·6 Noise problems

Many elderly people experience noise problems, particularly from neighbours, but sadly there are no easy solutions. Most difficulties can be resolved only through the goodwill of the people involved, and this is often in short supply. If you do want to pursue matters further there are certain steps you can take, but proving noise nuisance is notoriously difficult.

If you are a council or housing association tenant you should contact your housing manager. If he or she feels it would be helpful for the noise levels to be measured, arrangements can be made. If you are a private tenant or home owner you can contact the local council to ask an environmental health officer to visit your home and assess the extent of the problem. This of course means that the noise must be evident when the inspector is actually visiting, which is one reason why noise nuisance can be so difficult to prove.

A leaflet entitled *Bothered by Noise?* is available free from advice centres.

5·7 Help with heating

Age Concern England has specialist information both on financial help with heating costs and on ways of keeping warm. Fact sheet No. 1 *Help with Heating* is available free on receipt of a 9½" x 6½" SAE from the Information and Policy Department. It covers the following:

- Supplementary benefit, housing benefit and heating costs
- Insulation grants and improvement grants
- Easy ways to save energy

- Easier payment schemes for gas and electricity
- Disconnections
- Services provided by the Fuel Boards and assistance from social services
- Where to go for further help

There are now a large number of neighbourhood energy projects which can give advice and practical assistance to elderly people whose homes need insulating and draughtproofing.

*You can find out if there is an energy project in your area by writing to **Monergy Saver**, Freepost, Newcastle upon Tyne NE1 1BR. You do not need a stamp.*

5·8 Meeting your housing costs

There is not the space in this booklet to cover in any depth the different benefits and allowances which are available to elderly people in particular circumstances, but the Age Concern England booklet *Your Rights*, mentioned later, has full details. Also the welfare benefits system changes completely in April 1988, after which you should ensure that any information you are given is up-to-date. After that date supplementary benefit will become 'Income Support'.

Three aspects of the welfare benefits system relating to housing costs need to be highlighted here:

Housing benefit   The most important thing you should know is that if you do not currently receive housing benefit (ie help with rent and/or rates) and if you have not recently checked whether you are entitled to any help, you should consult a Citizens Advice Bureau or welfare rights advice centre. Housing benefit is administered by local councils, for the DHSS. Up to April 1988 a claim for housing benefit is assessed only on your income, with your savings not taken into account at all. From April 1988, though, people with savings of £3,000-£6,000 will get less housing benefit than they have been receiving up till then, and those with savings of more than £6,000 will no longer qualify for housing benefit.

Flat owners If you own a flat or any other property on a long lease, and are eligible for supplementary pension, you may be able to get an addition towards the weekly cost of your ground rent and service charges. Not all the elements of the service charge might be covered, the cost of window cleaning for example. This help may not be available after April 1988.

Help with removal costs If you qualify for supplementary pension and have only £500 savings or less, you may be able to get help with your removal costs. This assistance is in the form of a single payment, ie a grant from the DHSS, towards the cost of using a removals firm. You will have to get estimates and submit them to the local social security office for their approval *before* you hire a removal firm. You may also get a payment to cover your own travel costs to your new home on the day you move.

Elderly people in receipt of supplementary pension may be able to get a grant for essential basic furniture and £75 towards other essential household items if you do not have these already, possibly if you are moving from furnished to unfurnished accommodation. Grants can also be obtained for the cost of disconnecting and reconnecting your cooker and heating appliances when you move.

Help with removal costs may no longer be available after April 1988.

Further information The following Age Concern England fact sheets are available free on receipt of a 9½" x 6½" SAE from the Information and Policy Department:
No. 16 *Supplementary Benefit and Savings/Capital*
No. 17 *Housing Benefit*
No. 25 *Supplementary Benefit; Regular Weekly Income*

The Age Concern England booklet *Your Rights*, which is updated annually, describes all the main benefits and pensions for which elderly people may qualify, so that you can check you are claiming your full entitlement. It costs 90p from larger branches of W.H. Smith or from the Marketing Department of Age Concern England.

If you have any doubts about whether you qualify for a particular benefit, or problems with one you already get, you should contact a Citizens Advice Bureau or welfare rights advice centre.

USEFUL ADDRESSES

Age Concern England
60 Pitcairn Road
Mitcham
Surrey CR4 3LL
Tel: 01-640 5431

Age Concern Scotland
33 Castle Street
Edinburgh EH2 3DN
Tel: 031-225 5000

Age Concern Wales
1 Park Grove
Cardiff CF1 3BJ
Tel: 0222 371821

Age Concern Northern Ireland
6 Lower Crescent
Belfast BT7 1NR
Tel: 0232 245729

Centre on Environment for the Handicapped
35 Great Smith Street
London SW1P 3BJ
Tel: 01-222 7980

Disabled Living Foundation
380-384 Harrow Road
London W9 2HU
Tel: 01-289 6111

Housing Corporation
Head Office:
149 Tottenham Court Road
London W1P 0BN
Tel: 01-387 9466

Regional Offices:

London and Home Counties (South)
Pembroke House
Wellesley Road
Croydon
Surrey CR9 2BR
Tel: 01-681 3771

London and Home Counties (North)
Waverley House
7-12 Noel Street
London W1V 4BA
Tel: 01-434 2161

West
35A Guildhall Centre
Exeter EX4 3HL
Tel: 0392 51052/4

East Midlands
Phoenix House
16 New Walk
Leicester LE1 6TF
Tel: 0533 546762

West Midlands
Norwich Union House
Waterloo Road
Wolverhampton WV1 4BP
Tel: 0902 24654

North East
St Paul's House
23 Park Square South
Leeds LS1 2ND
Tel: 0532 469601

Merseyside
6th Floor
Corn Exchange Buildings
Fenwick Street
Liverpool L2 7RD
Tel: 051-236 0406

North West
Elisabeth House
16 St Peter's Square
Manchester M2 3DF
Tel: 061-228 2951

Wales
24 Cathedral Road
Cardiff CF1 9LJ
Tel: 0222 384611

Scotland
Rosebery House
9 Haymarket Terrace
Edinburgh EH12 5YA
Tel: 031-337 0044

SHAC
(The London Housing Aid
Centre)
189A Old Brompton Road
London SW5 0AR
Tel: 01-373 7276

Shelter
88 Old Street
London EC1V 9AX
Tel: 01-253 0202

INDEX